# Ward Rounds

# Ward Rounds

poems

K. Dale Beernink

GRAYSON BOOKS
West Hartford, Connecticut
graysonbooks.com

Ward Rounds
Published by Grayson Books
West Hartford, Connecticut
ISBN: 978-1-7364168-7-7
Library of Congress Control Number: 2021924970
3rd edition, 2022

Interior & Cover Design by Cindy Stewart
Cover Photo: amonphan comphanyo/Shutterstock.com

for Pat McKegney and Ralph Wallerstein
and
Margaret

without whom would not be
Hanna Marie

# Foreword

I met Dale Beernink at a New Year's Eve party in 1965. My medical school neighbors upstairs invited the guests, but we used my apartment because it was a few square feet bigger than theirs. I'd put out some unshelled nuts in a bowl, a wooden cutting board, and a hammer. Dale walked in and immediately engaged himself with the challenge of opening the nuts. And he asked, "Whose idea was this?"

A few days later, after I had already told my mother I'd met the man I was going to marry, Dale announced himself by doing a handstand on the railing by my front door. It was a whirlwind courtship during his final days of Stanford medical school. Within six months, we had married and moved to New Haven, Connecticut, where Dale had an internship in internal medicine at Yale-New Haven Hospital. He began his first daily rounds on July 1, 1965.

It was a difficult year with exhausting hours. I was a graduate student at Yale in Education and he seemed to live at the hospital. Sometimes he would leave on Friday morning and not return from the wards until Sunday evening. We did not connect Dale's extreme fatigue with illness until he had a blood test and was diagnosed with chronic myelocytic leukemia in May 1966. He was to live only three more years.

The process of writing *Ward Rounds* helped Dale deal with his own personal tragedy with courage and dignity. On the one hand, he recognized himself as a healer and observer, and on the other as patient. Intellectually, he enjoyed the discipline of composing in different verse forms and sharing his efforts with a neighborhood poetry group.

We had moved back to Palo Alto in the Fall of 1966 so that Dale could work a less demanding schedule, one that could flex as he underwent grueling chemotherapy treatments in 1968-69. He became a research fellow at Stanford Fleischman Laboratories and practiced his medical diagnostics doing physicals for new university employees.

Off work, he was a devoted husband and father. He also founded a local chapter of Physicians for Social Responsibility, played jazz trumpet with local enthusiasts, participated in amateur recorder groups, and took up new instruments, including the Baroque krummhorn and the bassoon. He built a harpsichord from a kit and gathered friends for a rousing Brandenburg Concerto in our living room.

The complex, gifted man I married, Kenneth Dale Beernink, was born in Holland, Michigan, in 1938. He graduated as valedictorian of his class at John Muir High School in Pasadena in 1956 and went on to earn both his undergraduate and medical school degrees at Stanford, where he was elected to the Phi Beta Kappa and Alpha Omega Honor Societies. Dale performed on the Stanford gymnastic team—hence, the handstand—and he led an amateur jazz group that played in off-campus venues.

During his tenure at medical school, Dale spent a year at the Pasteur Institute in Paris working on immunological research. He became fluent in French, bonded with his European colleagues through work and music, and met his Beernink ancestors in Holland.

Dale and his father published the first edition of *Ward Rounds* in 1968 for family and friends. After Dale's death in 1969 at the age of 31, Washington Square East Publishers issued a second edition of the book. Now, more than half a century later, thanks to Richard M. Ratzan, M.D., of the University of Connecticut School of Medicine, and Ginny Connors at Grayson Books, new readers will have access to these poems.

In honor of Dale's musical persona, I established the K. Dale Beernink, M.D. Memorial Scholarship for Trumpet at the San Francisco Conservatory of Music. Dale's family legacy lives on through our daughter Hanna, to whom he dedicated the first edition, and our three grandchildren.

Margaret Rose Beernink Badger
November 2021
Monterey, California

# Preface to First Edition

The hospital ward is a world unto itself, a world unknown to most people except for fleeting encounters with it at the extreme ends of their lives. Even patients with chronic diseases spend as little time as possible on the ward and prefer to forget their experiences there. The cooks, the laundry workers, the janitors, the switchboard operators, the aides, the dieticians, the nurses—all those who keep this world in order and operating smoothly—go home after eight hours a day to their own real worlds. Even the local private doctors, who populate the hospital ward with their patients, limit to a minimum the time they spend there.

But for the interns and resident physicians, the young men and women in white, the hospital is the real world where they work, eat, sleep, and sometimes relax. The rare hours they spend elsewhere are usually consumed by sleep. For these doctors, times of day become unimportant and seasons become periods of more or less likely admissions of pneumonias, myocardial infarctions or smoke inhalations. These young doctors must be the ones to tell the story of the hospital ward.

Although young physicians have a multitude of motives for wanting to wear the hospital white, and although they are hardly homogeneous in the degree of their idealism, nevertheless they all spend their intellectual (and most of their emotional) energy attempting to understand and improve the lot of sick people. In performing this task, they place high value on objectivity and "cultivating the art of detachment." Yet each is, perforce, a party to innumerable intimate relationships between himself, the patient and an illness.

Each doctor makes it his job to influence these triadic relationships— hopefully to the patients' advantage. In turn, each doctor is equally subject to being influenced by them. In the end, even the least sensitive physician is permanently marked by the years he spends on his hospital wards.

I have attempted in these pages to tell part of the story of the hospital ward in the form of a series of verses, each of which is complete as an isolated episode, just as each doctor-patient ward encounter is a unit of experience to the physician. Poetry in this case seems to me an appropriate form for a physician to use. Poems are made by men puzzling over the larger questions in life, questions often having to do with birth, death, suffering, and the meaningfulness of one man's relationship to another. Moreover, few men are as close as doctors to the naked physical aspects of these questions—their touch, smell, sound, feel, and appearance.

Yet this proximity of physicians to the raw ingredients of life and poetry has failed to produce a sizable corps of doctor-poets. Perhaps this is because the challenge put to the physician is not merely to phrase these larger questions nor to understand their implications, but to do something about them every working day. This leaves little time for poems.

Thus, it was during my own illness that I had the time to write these poems—a time when my own experiences as a medical student and a hospital "house officer" were still fresh in my memory. This was a time when my patients reappeared to me and I lived again in my mind all the many emotions we experienced together.

Taken separately each poem is a mosaic of factual details collected from many patients suffering from a given disease or condition, and a synthesis of my subjective reactions to them. Taken together, the poems comprise a poetic aspect of the larger picture of the hospital ward as seen by one who lived and learned in it.

K. Dale Beernink
January 1969
Palo Alto, California

# Contents

# Introduction

My well-worn copy of *Ward Rounds* has the date "October 19, 1970" written on the flyleaf in my 25-year-old hand. I was a fourth-year medical student at that time at Columbia Physicians & Surgeons, only a few months from graduation. I can't recall how Kenneth Dale Beernink and I met, but his book was to play an important role in my life. I instantly recognized it as a classic and one that spoke to me as someone who wanted to be both a physician and a writer. I returned to it often over the years. I always made sure I had it nearby. I still do.

The poems are spare, direct and use "my" language, i.e., "meningitis", "osteoarthritis" and "septicemia" without descending into jargon. They deal with people whose clinical entities I could recognize as a medical student, persons at the unique intersections of their illnesses and their emotions, social setting, and psychological make-up. In other words, each poem represents an individual, idiosyncratic person.

Years later, studying the poetry of William Carlos Williams, another physician poet, I was struck by the similarities of what Beernink and Williams had attempted in their poetry. In fact, Beernink's preface and William Carlos Williams's autobiography are mirrors of each other:

> Williams: There the thing was, right in front of me. I could touch it, smell it…. Oh, I knew it wasn't for the most part giving me anything very profound, but it was giving me terms, basic terms with which I would spell out matters as profound as I cared to think of.[i]

> Beernink: I have attempted in these pages to tell part of the story of the hospital ward in the form of a series of verses, each of which is complete as an isolated episode, just as each doctor-patient ward encounter is a unit of experience to the physician. Poetry in this case seems to me an appropriate form for a physician to use. Poems are made by men puzzling over the larger questions in life, questions often having to do with birth, death, suffering, and the meaningfulness of one man's relationship to another. Moreover, few men are as close as doctors to the naked physical aspects of these questions—their touch, smell, sound, feel, and appearance.[ii]

Besides a similar flair for incorporating the vernacular into these poetic set pieces, Beernink shares with Williams an interest in the glimpse, the glance that takes it all in, "in a flash," as Burke described the creative process of Williams. Indeed, both Beernink and Williams are what Kenneth Burke, the literary critic and lifelong friend of Williams, called "master(s) of the glimpse." [iii] Perhaps this is a talent physician-writers glean from their intense clinical one-on-one encounters, often compressed in the hustle and bustle of medicine.

Like Williams, Dr. Beernink wrote most of poems in free verse. But not always. For Dr. Beernink was a poet also interested in formal poetry. "Anonymous," a poem about spontaneous abortion, is a villanelle. A poetic form originating in 17th Century France, the villanelle, with its repetitive refrains, is a very effective form for emphasizing certain thoughts in the poem. The final haikus in the book are another example of Beernink's experiments with form, although a shorter form here based on syllables, not rhyme. Any reader who has ever been an intern, or near one, will appreciate these final haikus. I feel a certain gratitude that Dr. Beernink captured the way I felt many a long lonely evening with too many hours and patients to go before sunrise.

Yet the gratitude is bittersweet. Kenneth Dale Beernink's *Ward Rounds* was published months before his death in 1969 of chronic myelocytic leukemia. The collection was recognized as the work of a born poet. Sadly, his promise never had the opportunity to blossom further, since he died at the age of 31, three years after his diagnosis of a disease that now has a life-expectancy comparable to that of age-matched controls, that is, people without this disease. Incredibly, however, he was able, while undergoing chemotherapy for his leukemia and working as a research fellow at Stanford, to continue playing the cornet, to help raise a new baby daughter, build a harpsichord and write *Ward Rounds*.

His poems illuminate insights into the kinds of patients physicians and nurses encounter regularly. Beernink appreciated the irony in clinical medicine, saving for the last line of "Baby Thadeus Washington" the fact that, unbeknownst to the mother, her rubella eleven months earlier was the cause of her newborn's death. Thankfully few, if any, babies born in the U.S. since 1969, when the vaccine was introduced, are born with congenital rubella. The anachronistic medicine in *Ward Rounds* is one of its charms—its descriptions of illnesses and circumstances of medicine of a bygone era preserved in the amber of Dr. Beernink's verse.

*Ward Rounds* is a poetic time capsule we are opening fifty years after its first publication. It includes references to the kinds of patients medical professionals no longer see. For example, I distinctly remember memorizing, in the early 1970's, which barbiturates were short-acting and which were long-acting, both facts affecting our management of overdoses. More: my wife and I learned physical diagnosis in 1969, while Dr. Beernink was writing his lapidary poems, and patients with heart murmurs were staying for months or years in chronic disease hospitals, comforted by family photos and flowers. But the last barbiturate ingestion I saw was over 40 years ago. "Wards" and residential hospitals and a society that treated patients and medical students that kindly are of historical interest only—memories for the Smithsonian—extinct now, as extinct as the dodo, at least in this country. When one reads *Ward Rounds*, one is reading a poetic version of a 1969 Sears Roebuck Catalog.

*Ward Rounds* and its poet-physician, Dr. Kenneth Dale Beernink, who would be 83 as I write this in late 2021, deserve a newer, younger audience. I am very grateful to Dr. Beernink's widow, Margaret Rose Beernink Badger, and to Ginny Connors, the generous and wise publisher of Grayson Books, for making this publication possible, a full half century and more after its first edition.

Richard M. Ratzan
December 2021
West Hartford, Connecticut

---

[i] Williams, WC. *Autobiography.* New Directions; NY, 1951:357.

[ii] Beernink, KD. *Ward Rounds.* Second Edition. Washington Square East; Wallingford, PA; 1970.

[iii] Burke, K. "Sour Grapes," in: Doyle, Charles. William Carlos Williams: The Critical Heritage. London: Routledge & Kegan Paul, 1980: 70-73.

# Penny Brown

*rheumatic heart disease*

One other admission, at age eighteen,
Your record stated: normal labor,
Infant dead at birth. Between
Confinements you'd seen Hell and said,
"That's life." Your husband, sobbed your neighbor
Who'd accompanied you, "had led

A Christian life, but couldn't earn
No liven widout schoolin." You'd
Spent twenty barren years to learn,
At thirty-eight, you carried the child
He wanted long ago. Pursued
By creditors and age, he piled

His coveralls and married love
Into a sack and left to find
A welfare state where wives, above
All else, were had without the fear
Of hospital bills and babies combined.
Your neighbor lady made that clear.

I spent an extra hour with you
That night. Rheumatic heart had failed
At three full months. The rales, the grey-blue
Lips, the puffy legs—small hope
To live through labor. I detailed
To you the signs my stethoscope

Knew well. You thought that you'd done right
In spending all of last month's welfare
Check on baby clothes despite
The empty heart-pill bottle you'd
Been told could mean your life. No tear
Was spilled until I had renewed

My plea that you'd be saved no other
Way than by abortion. Trying
Hard to make you see another
Lighter side I blundered on
About your age disqualifying
You from motherhood. Upon

The name of baby Christ you swore
You'd kill yourself if that were true.
But not until the time you'd bore
That child, or died in bearing it.
I set your nasal cath, and drew
Your blood and knew that I'd permit

No scalpel to intrude between
Your baby and your being, in name
Of saving life. The strength I'd seen
In you I couldn't understand
As only blood and bone; in shame
Of preaching death I took your hand

And asked you what it was that cut
Your wind, a boy or girl. You smiled
Into my starched, white, world from what
Black-ghettoed, sickly ignorance
I couldn't guess. But great with child
You'd found your peace; no indigence

Or prejudice denied you this.
How then, could I? You sensed my pain
Despite the expressionless edifice
Of objectivity I'd built
To hold my sanity. Again
You smiled, and asked me if I'd tilt

Your bed a bit so you could see
The dime store crucifix that hung
Above.

The charge nurse called at three:
"She's gone—don't run." I rushed through sleep
To see your final smile, your lung
A mass of embolus. The cheap

Tin cross still fixed in your soft stare.
Surviving you, the fetus turned
Inside, and died, as unaware
Of birth in death as life. Your labor
Left you peaceful.

                    I returned,
Explaining "blood clot" to the neighbor.

# Stenton Brack

*manic psychosis*

Three pictures of yourself on your nightstand
Your silver star hanging from your polka-dot tie
And the suitcase full of inventions you insisted
Would be patented tomorrow but for lack of funds
And would I keep you in mind.

Three long weeks I never saw you sleep.
We walked my ward together during the smallest hours
And I grinned at your jokes and your clang associations
Though you never knew I did.
What several hours I slept that month I know the night crew
Watched you talking to the BIRDS and the I.V. stands
With ecstatic enthusiasm about your single-handed
      successes
On Iwo Jima.

And we fed you enough chlorpromazine to pacify
The population of all of New Haven
But still you paced and joked and laughed and offered,
Each morning, to give me your polka-dot tie.

When I transferred you to the incoming tern
My handwriting trembled on my "off-service" note
As I printed the diagnosis "Psychosis"
And wondered who was really sane.

# Bartholomew Stard

*traumatic decortication*

Always the blinds were pulled in your room where you waited,
Patient as a pupa, for a diaper change or a turn
Onto last week's bedsore. Your sightless eyes would burn
White in the dark while your soul crouched in the corner.

Monthly that winter your mother came and repeated
Her conviction that you, "would soon be looking better."
And proudly numbered the gooks you'd killed before
The shrapnel buried your mind in Asia's mud.

For a year synthetic life had been pumped to your blood
Through dozens of tubes. Each day the residents
Were pleased to see your heart and lungs were clear—
Organs serving no intelligence.

Then one morning we found your BIRD unplugged. The corner
Was empty. I opened the blinds. Spring was near.

# Jackson Spander

*acute and chronic bronchitis*

He hadn't the wits to show me signs
Like his friend had done
To convince me he was crazy enough to be committed,
Just for the winter.

He hadn't the courage to say he was famished,
That his bedsore was oozing stinking pus,
That he didn't have the strength to ride the boxcar
To Pensacola this year,
That he thought he was afraid of dying
On a park bench.

He didn't even know that he was asking me
To take care of him:
"Hell, Doc, I was takin care of myself
Before your daddy had fuzz on his chin!"
And when he laughed, he hacked his bloody phlegm
Through a toothless, smelly grin
And filled his paper cup.

But he spent that winter on my ward
In the V.A. hospital.

# Stanley Long

*barbiturate ingestion*

Brief encounter
Across the red blanket
Across a short score of years
For me to pronounce you
Officially finished in my thin black script
For some keeper of records
To fastidiously file.

>"Can't understand why a handsome kid..."
>Barked the driver of ambulances,
>Used to the stink of six-day old bodies.

I knew that you had bravely shared
His lack
Of understanding.

And I noted
Before I replaced your red shroud
That you'd neatly combed your hair
While you waited
To go
To sleep.

# Candy Den Blatt

*barbiturate ingestion*

From the county's north suburbs she came, carried by sirens
And wrapped in red lights, threatening to fall asleep
Threatening to snooze, to close her eyes, to take a long nap,
Though no one had heard her use the verb "to die."

In her red rayon, plunging night gown and blue painted eyes
She was better prepared than I for our encounter
At four A.M. and she swallowed the tube with a vigorous
Eager gulp, and she seemed to relish the retching.

At forty-three she had visited scores of physicians
Carried six diagnoses of psychosomatic disease
And a purse full of pills and prescriptions compounded to ease
Tension, depression, agitation, sleeplessness, and - much more.

Her husband came later, like a child who'd been whipped; trembling,
Defeated, repeating, "Will she be all right, Doc?"
But then not listening to my reply as if a lack
Of certainty was somehow very reassuring.

After sleeping all day, she awoke and repeated in triumph
How very close to death she was certain she'd been.
Then she left with a grin on the arm of her cowering man.
I ended her note with a question: *"Attempted suicide?"*

# Theodosus Bull

*delirium tremens*

You walked in off Howard
And told of two fifths a day
And we didn't believe you—
      Until you belched blood
          and the aide fainted.

And you wept dry tears
To see the technicolor worms
Shucking your skull like a rotten pecan
And we didn't believe you—
      Until you stuck your head
          through the window pane.

And you mumbled of rats and riots
And drinking after-shave lotion
And your kid in the can
And we didn't believe you—
      Until we scraped off your socks.

And you babbled on about
The injustices you'd suffered at the
Hands of society
And we didn't believe you—
      Until the night nurse found you hanging
          peacefully by your neck
          from the saliva aspirator.

# Janie McBride

*toxemia of pregnancy*

Only and much valued daughter
Of a rural chief of police
And sweetest of all the black-haired
Village ladies at seventeen.
Only one boyfriend and only one
Time on the seat of the Ford
With your lovely hair in a bun
Behind the gym and, "He's not
To know of his fatherhood,"
Was your black-eyed command.

Six months you deceived your plain parents
Confined in kimonos and bathrobes,
Your black hair fixing in curlers,
Smiling over breakfast at your father
And suffering each kick of your act
Of sin. Then they sent you up here
With their blessing, thinking you started
A virgin in business college
Where tuition was free.

      You sat
With the county's poor and dirty
Mothers attending the prenatal
Clinic. I never saw
You smile. The last month you swelled
In toxemia, but still you rolled
Your young black hair in Hollywood's
Latest styles, and rimmed
Your proud eyes with green. Then I suffered
Your labor, my hand on your pale
Stretched abdomen and protestant guilt-racked
Soul.

We delivered him breech,
And I sewed up a third-degree tear
With no whimpers. But you wept real tears
At the sound of his first strong cry
Then turned your head away
And bit your bleeding lips
And gave him to fortune and the county
Adoption agency.

.

When you left
Our post-natal clinic to find
A free business school, no green
Shadow rimmed your eyes
And your black hair was loose and shining
On your shoulders.

# Anonymous

*spontaneous abortion*

Quiet as blood was conception's act.
Whispered the first premonition that you had life;
And silent as love is your formless dying.

Cold as death was the surgeon's curette,
And cold were the starched white sheets which gave
        you greeting;
Though hot as this blood was conception's act.

Long were the hours a woman spent dreaming
Of long walks with a beautiful child, of long years of
        loving;
And brief as this night is your formless dying.

Slow is the healing to follow your fact,
And slow the forgetting of all you were to be;
Though hurried as blood was conception's act.

Joyous the woman who knew you were growing,
And cheerful with light were her days in the knowledge
        of you;
But black as despair is your formless dying.

Loudly this night sounds a woman's weeping,
And loud in its silence no infant is crying;
Though quiet as blood was conception's act
And silent as love is your formless dying.

# Baby Thadeus Washington

*rubella syndrome*

Burrowing blind in the bedclothes
Your eyes with cataracts
Were opaque as two shiny nickels
On your chubby black four-month-old face.

As I listened in trance
To the murmur of blood
Through the holes in your tiny sick heart
I saw your mama place a trembling hand on yours
And I wondered if she'd felt the least bit ill
When she erupted in German measles
Eleven months before.

# Baby Brenda Bulefsky

*failure to thrive*

Minikin skeleton stretched with rice-paper skin
In one hand I held you
A tissue and balsa creation
Tethered by tiny I.V. tubing
Tenuously placed in a thread-size vein on your scalp.

I transfused thimblefuls of blood
And when you'd taken thirty mils of milk by mouth
I watched the painful peristalsis
Pass beneath your navel like
A miniature bag of worms.
And I smiled when the nurses dubbed you "Tiger"
And taped a small pink bow atop
Your bald, translucent, six-week-old skull.

No one believed that your mother, just fifteen,
Loved you like her record collection,
Or that she had been trying to feed you
Hamburger
And beans.

And when you'd regained your birth weight
We taught her of milk and nipples and belches
And we discharged you into
A more gentle world.

# Child Tony Ribi

*septicemia*

You never saw my ward, contaminated
With the wrecks of adult excess, drink
Stained livers and smoke scored lungs. The stink
Of prodigal maladies, which saturated
My starched whites and even permeated
My stiff reason, never soiled your urchin
Nares, which moved no air while I was searching
For you through the E.R. where you waited.

"Fourteen, too old for pediatrics, Doc."
The medical resident said, "We've got to treat
Him here, then to your ward."

                    But his prediction
Never saw my ward; in septic shock
You shook life free determinedly, a feat
To teach my laggard moribunds conviction.

# Benjamin Scoggins

*rheumatoid arthritis*

He spent eight years watching his hands
Become claws, and waking in screams
When he turned on his hot, swollen knees
In his dreams, chasing the limber
Young man that he was in Soho.

He cursed my U.S. in his cockney
Accent, for the friends who deserted
Him, for his decomposed joints and the price
Of the prednisone, splints and x-rays.

When at last he'd been fired from his job
On the line, bankrupt and in tears
And unable to lift his dead arms
To dry his red-rimmed eyes
He accepted my thought that perhaps
He'd find peace and some comfort on National
Health, on the arthritis wards
Of London's Saint Bartholomew.

His postcard still hangs on my bulletin
Board with its bright Union Jack,
Big Ben, and "...wish you were here."

# Gino Spinelli

*acute lymphocytic leukemia*

"No next of kin," you'd said that night
They carried you onto my ward, but you smiled
At the grey-haired lady whose hand you held.
                                    Though I failed
That night to see her love for you, it wasn't long
Before you'd told us all that "you're as young
As you feel," and that's what made you feel like a child
Again, because you were in love.


                                    I paled
The color of my suit when first I heard
Your marriage plans. Unless the lab had erred,
You shouldn't have had the strength to grin
At me the way you did. Chaste
Mistress, Cancer, but she'd had her taste
Of the body you'd pledged to another.


                                    "So thin
He's gotten, Doctor; that must be what made him faint."

(Maria was certain that "thin" was "cause.")

                                    "Too bad things went
Like this, but we can wait till he gets out.
Been waiting all our lives for this, can wait
A little longer; haven't really set a date."


You'd spent your youthful energy on poverty,
The youngest of eleven in southern Italy,
And couldn't say hello in English when you arrived
At twenty-four, to find a fortune and some dignity.
They thought you always a fool, they contrived
Explanations for why you could not understand
The English too well, and why you would never demand

A higher price for a pound of tomatoes, and how
You could live through the New Haven winters alone
Without a regular job. Had they known
Of your loneliness would they have reasoned so?

You were cheerful as always the next Sunday morning.
You talked to the priest of Maria, and read him the sports page
And asked about all your old roommates.
                                        Your wheezing
Began after lunch, I recall. You sat on the edge
Of your bed trying so hard to smile, and explained
That your breathing was suddenly hard.
I could hear in your lungs what we all had feared,
And before I completed the cultures you leaned
On my shoulder—I saw that your smile had turned blue,
And quietly you
Convulsed.

I broke two of your teeth with the laryngoscope, but
In my fight to place the tube your cords stayed taut.
To the surgeon laryngospasm was nothing new,
And I helped him open your tubes too late
To mend your mind or move your sick white blood.
The nurses left and the priest arrived, and I made him wait
While I pumped your chest—
But your pupils never shrank.
                                        Quietly
He mumbled, "Doctor, you did your best."
And I gave you to him reluctantly.

I dialed the number for next of kin.
"Come right away, the turn is for the worse."
I fingered my sweaty lip and smelled
Your terminal vomitus. The day nurse
Shoved the death certificate before me, spelled
Your name in pencil, and left to join the outside world
Where life is three score and ten. I'd often called

To say the turn is for the worse—a deceit
To further compromise the already effete
Self-image of a healer that lay
Weeping in this wrinkled white.

But I had never called a fiancée.

# Morton Stump

*gout*

Your queen to be cushioned in fine silk pillows
And pampered like a pot of imported orchids—
She whom your mother once sweetly kissed and counted.
How she trembles now in the breath of your sighing
And flinches to think on the force of my awful whispers,
How she fills every sleeping corner of your dreams
With tumor and dolor.

For she has caused a proud man to weep,
She has caused a sane man to babble in delirium
And she has caused a strong man to tremble with pain—

Your hot, red, swollen, throbbing, hairy, left great toe.

# Minnie Freeme

*post necrotic cirrhosis*

Two volumes of medical record announced
That your comatose visit came almost monthly.
Paging through your paper existence I noted
The workups became progressively shorter, as is our habit,
Who think we know all after our first meetings.
I traced your social history back through dozens
Of epigrammatical *"see prior records"*
Until I came upon the yellowed page
And youthful pen of our first encounter with you,
Only to discover what I already thought I knew:

> *Patient totally deaf, lives alone, senile,*
> *No intelligent communication possible,*
> *Brought in by landlady whenever she becomes unresponsive.*

Poisoned by proteins, I explained once again to the kindly
Lady who brought you in. She seemed more concerned
About your hospital bill and how you'd ever pay
The rent, and why didn't your no-good daughters take you in,
And couldn't we keep you in the hospital this time?
But her tired smile said she'd never turn you out.

Two days of treatment and once again
You awoke to your soundless world and took some juice
And munched your toast
And smiled your gracious seventy years.
Though your case seemed pat
I requested the social service consultant
To see if society owed you anything,
Expecting to hear the reply, "No funds."

The day of your discharge I hurried the morning rounds
To your room where you sat in your all-purpose flower print
Fingering white knitted gloves, and wearing

A thirty-year-old hearing aid which, you explained
In lucid, Boston clipped tones, your doctor
(My social worker) had found in your tiny flat where it always
Got lost when your coma came on—and did I
Realize that today was Saint Valentine's Day?
(I, of course, did not.)

We helped you agree to a nursing home's care,
And before I dictated your chart I added a tiny
Red heart to the upper left corner of the *Social History*
That your real doctor had provided for you.
And my last progress note made the critical observation
On the change in your state of orientation:

> *This morning Mrs. Freeme has correctly informed us that*
> *Today is*
> *Saint Valentine's Day.*

# P. Fulton Dimmit

*senility*

They brought him from the farm in West County
When his soiling the bed every day
Made too much linen for the old washing machine
Now that his daughter's new baby arrived.

Searching for new conversation
When he'd been several weeks on my ward
I remarked on the pot of fresh rose buds
That always guarded his wrinkled form.

For an instant he seemed to grow younger
As a memory swelled in his throat,
"In my garden I'd let them die right on the plant,
It's so much better for the roots."

# Silas Gill

*osteoarthritic cervical spurring*

This time they found you on the street
Bawling that you couldn't walk,
A sixty-eight-year-old, white-haired baby.
They'd heard that before, but never in the summer
When street sleeping was good.
So they threw you, your bottle, and your tears
In the paddy.

"Doc, we were gonna keep him in a cell
But thought you aughta take a look."
Knowing the sergeant's habits
I knew this to mean that you were
Making too much noise in jail.

You had very good reason to bawl.
Three plus knee jerks and wasted quads;
From the films of your neck, it was hard to see
How anything could pass from your skull to your legs,
And we transferred you to neurosurgery.

In a short three weeks after cutting
You walked off the ward with a limp,
Twirling your cane.
I returned your wink and knew
That when I saw you next winter
I'd listen with care to every one
Of your noisy complaints.

# Johny Trummel

*Bright's disease*

Every day the musicians came
To fill your small room with their grinning
To lean on your bed where you sat
Propped up like a small wrinkled monkey,
Grey from your kidney's failings,
Babbling insane with the sickness
And wise in the knowledge of dying.

They came with their flowers and candy
To pay their respects to the drummer
Who'd joined all their spirits in rhythms
From New Orleans to Chicago.
They came with great boxes of records
To play back your finest percussion;
Some even appeared with their horns
Shrouded in black velvet cases
Their tuxedoes bare at the elbows,
For they were to play that same evening
At one-night stands in the city
And cry through their horns about Johny.

The walls had been long since covered
With photos of all the great bands
That had ever blown jazz to a crowd,

And somewhere in each of the photos
Your simian grin was propped
Behind bass, snares, and top hat cymbals

And your long electric fingers
Glinted black on the sticks.
There, at the head of your bed,
Was the finest portrait of all:
Arm in arm you all stood squinting

In front of the Eiffel Tower
Clad in your matching red blazers
With tiny American flags
On each black shining lapel—
And the signature scrawled with a pencil,
*"For Johny—Good Times—The Duke."*

All of them asked me to cure you,
All of them knew that I couldn't,
But none of them knew of my longing
To speak with them all of your dying
Through the jazz of a cornet's dark thirds.

You laughed with them all through the daylight
To the clatter of top-hats and rimshots.
But the nights you cried out at the darkness
Alone in your dwindling rhythms.
Then high in my room I'd imagine
Your trembling wrinkled black form
Stretched taut on the starched white sheets
In the cone of the night-light's white glaring.

Then once I came down through the dim,
Through my ward's last midnight whimperings
To stand in the dusk of your life
At the edge of the bedlamp's glaring
That caged your month-long ending.

But black in the nights of your dying
The walls were the end of existence
Where only the night-light's round image
Shone bright from each glassy photo
To multiply all of your trembling
Into thousands of tiny glitters
In the contracting time of your rhythms.

In thousands of night-light glitters
Containing your stellate form

Stretched black on that field of white
So small beside you I stood
In those thousands of glossy reflections.

Suddenly gone were the photos.
The walls disappeared in the void.
Our thousands of tiny reflections
Were thousands of glittering eyes
Of all the time's finest black jazzmen
Standing to pay you a tribute
In the night of your faltering rhythm.

Then all those musicians' bright eyes
Came alive in the night of your drumming,
Came wild in the night of your rhythms;
Deep in the black blew a cornet.
Then loud in the dark came the wailing.
The eyes squinted shut from the sweating
And all the walls trembled in rhythm
To the pounding of black jazzmen's feet
And the tubas bellowed progressions
Of generations of grieving
While the trombone slides flashed red
In the echo of your final cadence
Till the rumbling walls were an organ

Of New Orleans' laughing and sobbing
As hundreds of swaggering marchers
Tramped their brass through the night of your rhythm
And sweat in the beat of your drumming.
Their souls became sound in their horns
As they screamed your great joys and great sorrows.

There I floated in white on black sound
And my speech was a silver cornet
Half-valving the thirds and the sevenths
Muted with red rubber plungers
And growling my knowledge of dying

Through the coils of sweat stained silver
In the thundering of lifetimes of rhythms.

Then the music was gone—I was weeping.
And the eyes became night light's glittering
On dozens of glossy photos
Where your cruciform black was reflected
And I stood so small beside you
So small and alone beside you
In thousands of glittering reflections.

You were babbling insanely in the night,
Wise in the knowledge of dying.
So I left you alone with your rhythms.

# Jemimah Dill

*infectious mononucleosis*

Pale, thin and nervous you came with your husband.
Bibles in hand, biting your thin Baptist lips
In fear that your illness was sign of your God's last calling.

He told me how his dear old mother had sickened like you
Then died of a cancer and left him to Grandma in Georgia,
And he excused himself as he wept in anticipation

And planned aloud how he would set up his mission
Alone in the African jungle without your sweet presence,
(And was I aware that you were his model of goodness?)

I suggested the signs weren't too good—he decided the worst.
He explained how he, like old Job, would be tried by the loss
Of you, the thing he loved most in his life (after God).

When I told him it might not be nearly so bad as he thought
He assured me this world was full of the devil's worst evils
And not to be understood by preachers or doctors.

Then our lab tests disclosed you did not have malignant disease!
The mono would soon go away, I assured your young preacher,
So you would be free to move to a Gold Coast mission

To preach your firm faith to the naked black civilizations
And raise thin-lipped children to know how to recognize sin.
Without smiling he knelt at your bedside and read out of Job.

And I couldn't help seeing a passage he'd marked up in red:
        *"But when I looked for good, evil came,*
        *And when I waited for light, darkness came."*

And I wondered if he wasn't disappointed.

Then you walked off the ward hand in hand, pale, thin and nervous,
And alert for the very first signs of evil and darkness.

# Maxine Pick

*exogenous obesity*

Frightened by shortness of breath
And pains in her chest when she walked,
She checked in at three hundred thirty-five pounds
To spend six weeks on vitamin pills
And celery
And tea.

For three weeks she sulked in depression
Though she lost a pound every day,
So we gave her a pass to go home for Thanksgiving
With strictest prescription she eat only vitamin pills
And celery
And tea.

She returned the next morning
With a mysterious, satisfied smile
That stayed on her face for the last three weeks
Of her starvation diet of vitamin pills
And celery
And tea.

But she always changed the subject
When we asked her what was special about
The Thanksgiving vitamin pills
And celery
And tea.

# Violet Euridice Fontaine

*aseptic meningitis*

In an aura of steam and brown soap
You ascended from out of the laundry
With headache, stiff neck, and a chill,
Requesting we don't use no needles.

How could I grant your request?
In febrile prostration you suffered
The punctures, quietly defiant
So as not to be quietly fearful.

Our treatment was symptomatic.
Lacking good diagnosis
We first tried to do no harm,
Though you were convinced we were healing.

You improved in the hospital, just
As you would have at home, and you blessed
Us all with your primal smile
For draining the headache with needles.

On the seventh day you descended
Back into the laundry where work,
Not waiting, was the measure of men.
When I followed, a pale, starched Orpheus,

To pick up my weekly whites,
I saw your black-rimmed smile
Through the steam of a shirt pressing rig
Reminding me not to look back.

# Hospital Haiku

The new interns
        Stiff in starched white suits
The July heat!


Grinning into
        The newborn nursery
A man holding daisies.


Screaming objections
        In the hospital lobby—
A small naked boy.


All night below zero,
        Today in the clinic
New complaints of chest pain.


Resting on the stairs
        An old man with a large chest
And a cigarette.


Holding daffodils
        Near the hospital florist—
An old woman, weeping.


Only one room is lit
        In the hospital tonight—
And the August moon!

Beside this death bed
       Two old men
Embracing.

# Notes on the poems

The patients described in the poems are composites of many patients; the names assigned to them are inventions of the author.

## Penny Brown

Rheumatic heart disease can follow streptococcal disease. With the advent of antibiotics and widespread recognition of this cause-and-effect sequence, it has become very uncommon in the U.S.

Cath. refers to a small catheter with two prongs, one for each nostril, to deliver oxygen.

Mass of embolus refers to blood clots that originate elsewhere, usually the legs, which can break off and travel to the lung, where they can cause trouble breathing or even death. It is a dreaded event that can occur in pregnancy.

## Stenton Brack

BIRDS: This is a now-obsolete machine used to help a patient breathe without having to insert a tube into the trachea.

Tern is short for intern.

## Bartholomew Stard

Decortication is a devastating injury to the brain, leaving the person irreversibly unconscious.

## Candy Den Blatt

In this poem, "tube" refers to a nasogastric tube inserted into the stomach through the mouth (or nose) and esophagus, used for emptying the stomach of pills and for providing a conduit for irrigation of the stomach and its contents.

## Theodosus Bull

Delirium Tremens is a dangerous state of confusion and agitation following cessation of alcohol in some chronic alcoholics who abruptly stop drinking. It is often accompanied by hallucinations, seizures, and trembling.

Howard: In this poem Howard refers a street in New Haven, Connecticut, near the hospital where Dr. Beernink did his internship and residency.

## Janie McBride
Toxemia is a dangerous condition that can develop in pregnancy. It may present with a wide range of symptoms, from high blood pressure to seizures.

Third-degree tear: This refers to a ripping of the tissue around the vagina that can occur during the delivery of a baby, either as a result of the delivery or from an intentional cut in order to allow a wider opening for the baby to be born, sometimes needed for breech deliveries.

## Baby Thadeus Washington
Rubella syndrome: If a pregnant woman develops rubella (German measles), complications can occur in the infant, especially if the illness occurs during the first 12 weeks of gestation. Possible consequences include cataracts, congenital heart disease, and hearing impairment.

## Child Tony Ribi
Septicemia is the result of an infection, usually bacterial, that enters the blood stream. It can cause major disturbances such as dangerously low blood pressure and sometimes, as in this case, death.

Nares refers to nostrils.

## Benjamin Scoggins
Rheumatoid arthritis: Until the advent of the immunomodulators, rheumatoid arthritis was often a progressively deforming disease.

## Gino Spinelli
A laryngoscope is an instrument used to hold the mouth open and the tongue down while inserting a tube into the trachea in order to maintain the airway and provide mechanical breathing for the patient.

## Morton Stump
Gout: This metabolic disease is caused by excess uric acid. It primarily affects the kidneys and the joints, especially the big toe.

Tumor and dolor: These are two of the five markers of inflammation. In Latin, tumor refers to swelling and dolor refers to pain.

## Minnie Freeme
Poisoned by proteins: A cirrhotic liver has a very decreased ability to break down proteins normally produced by the body, leading to an accumulation of ammonia. This causes severe mental changes, primarily confusion and, ultimately, coma. Such mental changes are often reversible, as in this patient, with correction of the ammonia level.

## Silas Gill
Osteoarthritic cervical spurring: Arthritis can lead to abnormal bone formation that often takes the shape of spurs, which can, in the neck, interfere with nerves exiting the spinal cord. Pain and disability are the result.

Three plus knee jerks and wasted quads: These are signs of neurological impairment, in this case coming from higher in the spinal cord as a result of the interference of nerve impulses by the arthritic spurs in the neck. The knee jerks are deep tendon reflexes and wasted quads are quadriceps muscles that have atrophied from lack of nerve supply and use.

From your skull to your legs: The bony overgrowths had narrowed the space through which nerves and their impulses had to pass.

Cutting: In this poem cutting refers to the operative trimming away of any bony encroachment on nervous structures.

## Johnny Trummel
Bright's Disease was the term for what we now know is a large group of heterogeneous diseases causing glomerulonephritis, an inflammation of the glomerulus, the microscopic beginning of the filtration system in the kidney.

## Violet Euridice Fontaine
The Euridice in her name is a reference to a mythological figure. In the myth, after Euridice died, her lover Orpheus was allowed to attempt to bring her back from Hades on the condition of not turning around to see her following him while still exiting Hades. However, he gave into temptation and looked back.

Aseptic meningitis is a non-bacterial (aseptic) infection of the covering of the brain and spinal cord. It is usually caused by a virus.

To do no harm is a reference to medicine's age-old injunction in Latin, "Primum non nocere," which means "First, do no harm."

CPSIA information can be obtained
at www.ICGtesting.com
Printed in the USA
LVHW022356080222
710545LV00010B/644